Who Says 50 Can't Be Fabulous?

Stay Strong, Radiant, and Energized at Home

A Guide for Women 50+
to Stay Fit, Healthy, and Vibrant

By

J Vijaya

Qurate
quratebooks.com

Who Says 50 Can't Be Fabulous?
J Vijaya

Published in 2025
© Published by

Qurate Books Pvt. Ltd.
Goa 403523, India
www.quratebooks.com
Tel: 1800-210-6527, Email: info@quratebooks.com

ISBN: 978-93-5898-335-7

About the Author

Vijaya is a retired bank employee who discovered a vibrant new chapter in life after 50. When both her daughters moved away after marriage and she began facing menopausal challenges, aches, and emotional lows, she realized it was time for a change. With dreams long set aside due to family responsibilities, she decided to reclaim her energy and purpose. Inspired by supportive friends and social media, she began a soulful journey of self-renewal—staying active, listening to her heart, and fulfilling long-held aspirations.

Her debut book, Who Says 50 Can't Be Fabulous?, is a heartfelt reflection of that journey. Blending personal experience, storytelling, and practical wisdom, Vijaya encourages women to embrace self-care, vitality, and confidence—right from the comfort of home. She believes midlife is not an end, but a fabulous new beginning.

Contents

Introduction: Embracing Your Fabulous 50s and Beyond

"Who Says 50 Can't Be Fabulous?"

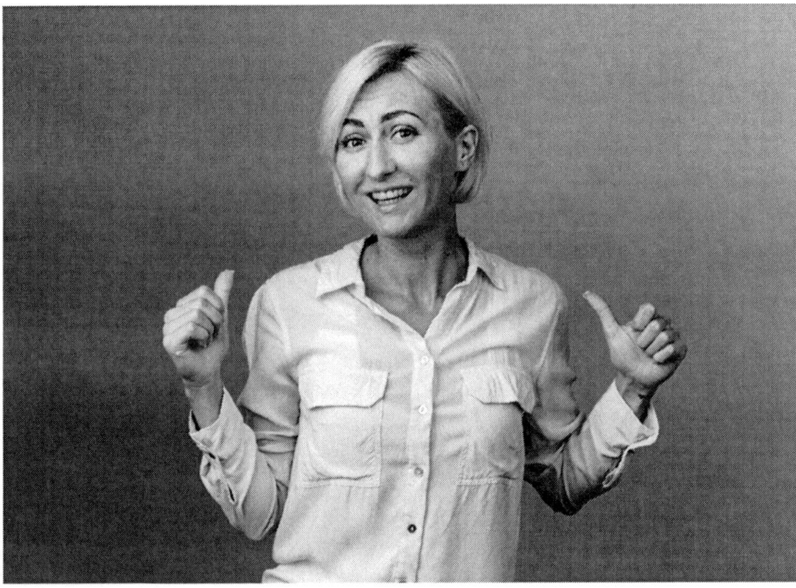

1: The Mindset Shift: Aging as an Opportunity, not a Limitation

For years, society has whispered—and sometimes shouted—that life slows down after 50. That energy fades, beauty diminishes, and dreams should be tucked away. Women are often told to shrink into the background, to retreat quietly, to make room for the younger generation.

But what if everything you've been told about aging is wrong?

What if your 50s—and every decade after—are your time to rise, to shine, to explore, and to expand?

What if, instead of shrinking, you bloom?

This book is your invitation to a new beginning. A beginning that starts not with a dramatic change in appearance or lifestyle—but with a deep, powerful shift in mindset, energy, and self-love. Whether you're 50, 60, or even 70+, your body and mind still carry the potential to glow with strength, purpose, and vitality.

"At 50, we don't fade—we focus."

2: Common Myths About Women Over 50 and Why They're Wrong

When you hit 50, things do change—let's not pretend otherwise. You might notice: Achy joints

- Stubborn weight gain
- Shifts in mood or motivation
- Sleep patterns that are not what they once were
- Hormonal changes that play hide and seek with your emotions

And yet, amid all this, there's a surprising gift: clarity. You begin to see what truly matters. You learn to say "no" without guilt. You begin to crave more meaning, more joy, and more connection. This phase is not about decline—it's about refinement. You're no longer chasing approval. You're seeking alignment—with your values, your passions, and your well-being.

"This is not about perfection—it's about participation in your own well-being."

3: Why Staying Active and Energized at Home Matters

If you're a woman at home, this book is especially for you.

Perhaps you're retired or nearing it. Maybe your children have grown up and moved out. Or you're busy taking care of grandchildren, elderly parents, or your home. You might have paused your career or changed your lifestyle.

Whatever your circumstance, one thing is true: you give. A lot.

This book is your reminder to also give—to yourself.

If you've ever:

- Looked in the mirror and wondered where your glow went
- Felt tired just getting through the day
- Questioned whether you're doing enough for your body or mind
- Thought it was "too late" to try something new

Then you're exactly where you need to be.

Sometimes, staying at home can feel isolating. It may seem like the world is racing ahead, and you're stuck in routines. But the truth is—this can be your most expansive season.

Imagine waking up with energy. Imagine enjoying your meals without guilt. Imagine looking forward to your mornings because they begin with joyful movement. Imagine your evenings filled with calm, laughter, or creativity.

You give so much. Now it's time to give to yourself—your strength, your peace, your joy.

"All this is possible. Not because of magic—but because of mindful, consistent action."

4: What to Expect from This Book

Why this book? Why now?

Because too many women spend this beautiful stage of life feeling invisible, exhausted, or unmotivated. And it doesn't have to be this way.

Because YOU matter. Your health, your dreams, your peace of mind, your sparkle.

I wrote this book because I know what it feels like to ask, "What now?" To feel the heaviness of change and wonder how to hold on to joy, purpose, and energy. And I also know the magic that happens when you start saying "yes" to yourself again.

This book is born from:

- My own journey of rediscovery at 50+
- The women I've met—friends, sisters, mentors—who inspired me with their stories of strength
- The challenges I faced and overcame with small, sustainable changes

Through experience, observation, and deep reflection, I've crafted this guide to support women like you—to remind you that your body is still a source of strength, your mind a wellspring of creativity, and your heart an endless reservoir of love.

You'll Discover:

1. Simple Home Workouts

No gym memberships. No intimidating equipment. Just easy movements you can do in your bedroom, balcony, or garden. From gentle yoga to strength training with water bottles, you'll discover how movement can be medicine.

2. Nutrition That Nurtures

Your body deserves nourishment that energizes, heals, and comforts. You'll learn how to create balanced meals, understand key nutrients for women over 50, and explore Indian recipes that are both delicious and healing.

3. Mindset Shifts for Confidence

Doubt is normal. So is growth. We'll explore how to replace old beliefs with new affirmations and how to rewire your thoughts to support your best self.

4. Stress Management and Emotional Wellness

With guided breathing, journaling, rest practices, and real stories from other women, you'll learn to navigate the emotional waves of life with more ease and grace.

5. Beauty and Self-Care from Within

Because feeling radiant isn't about looking younger—

it's about looking at yourself with kindness. Skincare, dressing up at home, sleep rituals, and confidence-building practices will help you glow.

6. Inspiration from Real Women

Throughout the book, you'll read real-life stories—of women who began businesses in their 60s, picked up old hobbies, healed from grief, and built new friendships.

Who This Book Is For

This book is for you if:

- You're a woman 50 or older who wants to feel better, think clearer, and live brighter
- You want to make changes but don't know where to start
- You're looking for practical advice, not perfection
- You want to be stronger, more peaceful, and more joyful
- You're ready to prioritize yourself without guilt

Whether you're just starting your wellness journey or reigniting a long-forgotten spark, this guide meets you where you are—with compassion and clarity.

This Is Your Time. Own It.

You are not too old. You are not too late. You are not done.

You are just getting started.

Each chapter is designed to encourage you to:

- Wake up with purpose
- Move your body with love
- Eat with mindfulness
- Think with clarity
- Rest with intention
- Glow with grace

Who says 50 can't be fabulous?

No one. Not anymore. Not here.

So, open your heart. Open your mind. Open this book—and let your most vibrant, radiant, confident chapter begin.

Because the best part of your life isn't behind you.

It's waiting for you.

Right now!

■ ■ ■

Chapter 1: The Foundation – Cultivating a Vibrant Mindset

"You are never too old to set another goal or to dream a new dream." — C.S. Lewis

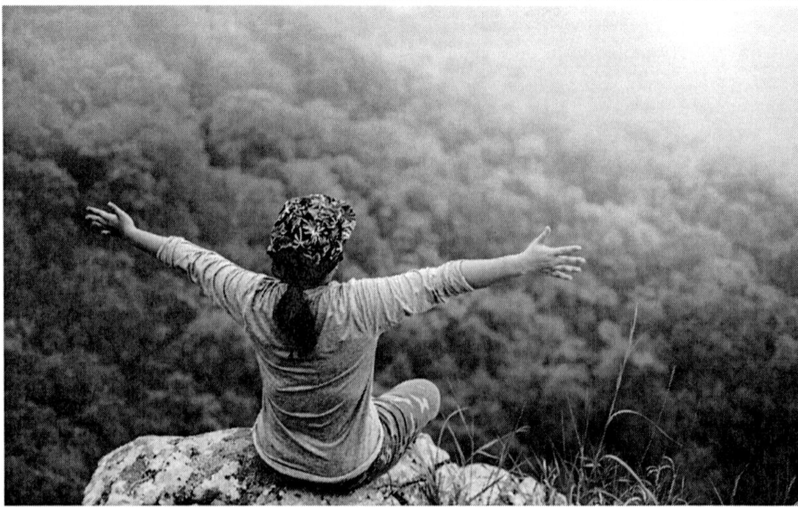

A New Chapter, A New You

Turning 50 is not the end of something—it is the elegant beginning of everything you still dream of becoming. For many women, this phase brings quieter mornings, empty nests, and changing roles. But rather than mourning what's gone, imagine this time as an invitation to rediscover your spark, nourish your soul, and fall in love—with yourself.

At 50 and beyond, you possess a treasure chest of life lessons, resilience, and grace. You've spent decades giving—now, it's your time to receive. To step back into the spotlight. To breathe deeply, live fully, and glow freely.

My Own Awakening: A Melody from Within

When I turned 52, the vibrant energy of my home shifted to a gentle hush. My children had flown the nest, and the silence echoed louder than I expected. I began to question—Where had I gone in all these years of caring for others? One evening, scrolling online, I found an ad for a virtual music class. My heart skipped a beat. I had loved singing as a girl, but life had put that passion on hold.

I signed up. I was nervous. My voice trembled in the first class. But over time, I began to sing—not just with my voice, but with my spirit. That one decision brought back color to my days. It reminded me: Passions don't age, they just wait patiently for your return.

1: The Power of Self-Belief and Positive Thinking

"Whether you think you can, or you think you can't —you're right." — Henry Ford

---

Your beliefs are the foundation of your reality. The story you tell yourself about aging becomes your truth. If you say, "I'm too old," your actions shrink. But if you say, "This is my time," you create magic.

Mindset Shift: Breaking Free from Limiting Beliefs

We grow up with beliefs like:

"It's too late to start something new."

"I don't have the energy anymore."

"People won't take me seriously at this age."

But these are not facts—they're just old stories. And the good news? You can rewrite them.

"It's not the years in your life that count.
It's the life in your years." – Abraham Lincoln

One powerful way to break through these limiting beliefs is through visualization. Close your eyes and imagine the woman you want to be—vibrant, energetic, joyful. Feel her presence. Speak as if she's already within you—because she is.

A Tale of Two Mindsets

Let's meet two women, both 50.

Sarah believes she's fading into the background. She talks about her aches and avoids mirrors. She stops trying new things.

Rita believes 50 is her rebirth. She signs up for drama classes, rediscovers painting, and surrounds herself with vibrant friends. Her eyes sparkle. She stands tall.

They are the same age. But their mindsets shape two entirely different realities.

Which one will you be?

The Science of Positive Thinking

Studies have shown that positive thinking isn't just about feeling good—it has real physical benefits. Women with an optimistic mindset:

✓ Live longer and have a lower risk of chronic diseases

✓ Experience less stress and more emotional resilience

✓ Are more motivated to stay active and take care of their health

Neuroscience supports this too. Positive thoughts release dopamine and serotonin—happy chemicals that improve mood, energy, and even immunity. Your thoughts are not just feelings—they are chemistry.

Real-Life Inspiration: Meena's Story

Meena, 53, used to wake up every day feeling tired and uninspired. She had convinced herself that her body was "too old" to exercise and that aging meant slowing down. But after a close friend introduced her to positive affirmations, everything changed.

She started each morning by saying:

✓ "I am strong, healthy, and full of energy."

✓ "I deserve to take care of myself."

✓ "Every day, I am becoming better and stronger."

Within weeks, she noticed a shift—not just in her mindset but in her actions. She started walking more, eating better, and feeling happier. All because she changed her thoughts.

Now, it's your turn. What is one positive belief you can adopt today?

Also try placing uplifting quotes on your mirror, fridge, or journal. Your environment can reinforce your empowerment.

2: Overcoming Self-Doubt and Embracing Confidence

"Confidence is not 'they will like me.' Confidence is 'I'll be fine if they don't.'" — *Christina Grimmie*

Many women over 50 grapple with self-doubt. We've been told our value declines with age, our beauty fades, and our purpose diminishes. But this is the time to rise, not retreat.

Confidence is not a personality trait—it's a practice.

How to Build Confidence After 50

✓ Acknowledge your achievements – You've raised families, built homes, supported others. That takes strength.

✓ Challenge Negative Thoughts: Replace "I'm not good enough" with "I am learning and growing every day."

✓ Dress for Success—Even at Home: Wear clothes that make you feel good.

✓ Try Something New: Stretch your comfort zone and grow.

✓ Surround yourself with positive people: Energy is contagious.

✓ Speak kindly to yourself: Would you talk to your best friend the way you talk to yourself?

"I am not afraid of storms, for I am learning how to sail my ship." – Louisa May Alcott

---

Confidence grows when you honor your own voice. Speak up in group chats, share your opinion, and don't apologize for taking space. You belong here.

Real-Life Inspiration: Rekha's Story

Rekha, 56, always wanted to dance but thought she was "too old to start." One day, she signed up for an online dance class. At first, she felt awkward, but as she practiced, she gained confidence—not just in dancing, but in life.

She realized that confidence isn't about being the best. It's about having the courage to try.

Rekha now mentors other women in her community, showing that age is no barrier to creativity or courage.

What's something you've always wanted to do but felt hesitant about?

Write it down. Then, take one small step toward it this week.

3: Daily Habits to Boost Motivation and Joy

"Small habits make big changes."

Joy isn't something you wait for—it's something you create every single day.

Simple Daily Habits

- ✓ Stretch each morning for 10 minutes – Boosts energy and mood.

- ✓ Dress up, even at home – Wear that lipstick. Drape that saree.
- ✓ Listen to music – Let melodies elevate you.
- ✓ Step outside – Fresh air and sunlight are nature's medicine.
- ✓ Talk to someone who makes you laugh – Connection keeps you youthful.
- ✓ Write down one thing you're proud of – Affirm your journey.

Also try:

- ✓ Drinking warm lemon water to start your day hydrated
- ✓ Lighting incense or essential oils that calm your mind
- ✓ Doing a "5-minute declutter" to bring clarity and order

Real-Life Inspiration: Priya's Story

Priya, 52, struggled with motivation. She felt drained every morning. But she started a simple morning routine:

1. 5 minutes of deep breathing
2. 10 minutes of light stretching
3. Writing one positive affirmation

This small change transformed her day. She had more energy, less stress, and a greater sense of purpose.

Now, she also leads a small morning WhatsApp group where women share affirmations daily.

Which of these habits can you start today?

Even just one can make a ripple through your entire day.

4: The Role of Gratitude and Mindfulness in Staying Vibrant

"Gratitude turns what we have into enough."
– Melody Beattie

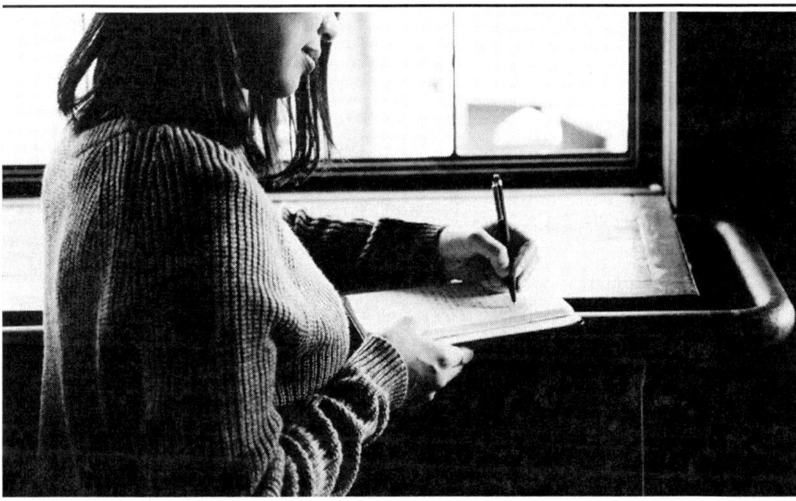

Gratitude and mindfulness are two simple yet powerful tools that can completely shift your energy and perspective.

Simple Ways to Practice Gratitude

- Start your day by listing 3 things you're thankful for.
- Keep a gratitude journal.

- Some days it may be big—your health, your home. Other days it's as simple as a good cup of chai or the scent of rain.
- Leave thank-you notes for loved ones. Tell yourself what you appreciate about you.

Practicing Mindfulness at Home

You don't need an ashram to be mindful. Just be present in your daily life:

✓ Sip your tea slowly, savoring every drop

✓ Feel the warmth of the sun on your skin

✓ Notice the rustle of leaves outside your window

✓ Take 5 deep breaths when you feel overwhelmed

✓ Light a candle and sit in silence for 5 minutes

Even cooking can be mindful—chopping vegetables with awareness, stirring gently, savoring the aromas.

Real-Life Inspiration: Anjali's Story

Anjali, 58, found herself constantly worrying about the future. She started a simple mindfulness practice:

Every morning, she wrote one thing she was grateful for. Every evening, she spent five minutes focusing on her breath.

Within weeks, she felt more at peace, more joyful, and more alive.

She also began painting simple mandalas as a meditative activity—and now shares them online, inspiring other women to pause and create.

What's one small act of gratitude you can do right now?

Pause and thank your body, your breath, your life.

Final Thoughts: Your Mindset is Your Power

This is your season to shine.

You've spent years nurturing others—it's time to nurture you. You are wise, strong, beautiful, and full of life.

Let go of doubt. Embrace your passions. Dance, laugh, love, and live out loud.

"And the day came when the risk to remain tight in a bud was more painful than the risk it took to blossom." – Anaïs Nin

---

Key Takeaways:

✓ Your mindset is your superpower. Think vibrant, age radiant.

✓ Confidence is built, not born. Start with small, brave steps.

✓ Joy is a choice. Make it daily.

✓ Gratitude and mindfulness can transform your days.

✓ You are not too old—you are right on time.

Your Action Steps:

✓ Start each morning with a positive affirmation.

- ✓ Take one small step outside your comfort zone this week.
- ✓ Keep a gratitude journal for the next 7 days.

Your 50s and beyond are not a time to slow down—they're a time to shine. By cultivating self-belief, confidence, joy, and gratitude, you set the foundation for a vibrant, energetic, and fulfilling life. Your mindset is your most powerful tool. Use it wisely, and watch how your life transforms.

The journey has just begun. And my friend, you are just getting started.

■ ■ ■

Chapter 2: Move It or Lose It – The Importance of Staying Active

"Take care of your body. It's the only place you have to live." – Jim Rohn

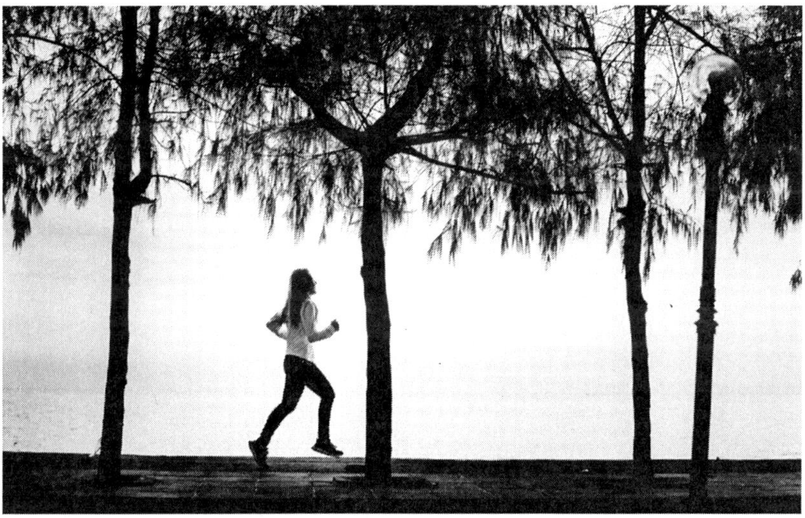

A Wake-Up Call: My Personal Story

It began with a dull ache in my knees. I brushed it off, assuming it was just part of aging. But soon, even climbing a few steps left me breathless. One evening, I found myself sitting alone after a long day, physically drained and mentally foggy. That was my moment of truth—I had slowly allowed myself to become inactive.

Everything changed when I visited a friend who radiated energy and positivity. She looked refreshed and graceful. Curious, I asked, "What's your secret?" Her answer was simple but powerful—movement.

She shared her daily morning routine:

1. Wake up at 6:30 AM
2. Five minutes of deep breathing
3. A glass of warm water with lemon
4. Gentle stretches with devotional music
5. Fifteen-minute indoor walk or terrace stroll

Inspired, I started small. Five minutes of stretches, followed by mindful breathing. Gradually, I added walking, a few strength exercises, and finally joined an online class tailored for women over 50. The transformation was slow but magical. My energy returned. My confidence grew. My smile came back.

Movement, I realized, isn't just about fitness. It's about reclaiming our lives.

1: Why Movement Matters More After 50

As we age, muscle mass naturally declines, bone density reduces, and flexibility diminishes. But these changes are not irreversible. Staying active can help prevent and even reverse many of these effects.

Benefits of Regular Movement:

✓ Strengthens muscles and bones

✓ Improves balance and reduces risk of falls

✓ Enhances heart health and regulates blood sugar

✓ Boosts mood, clarity, and emotional resilience

✓ Promotes better sleep and hormonal balance

"If you don't move it, you lose it."

Movement improves lymphatic circulation, reducing the risk of inflammation and supporting immune health. Regular physical activity also promotes the release of endorphins—the body's natural mood lifters.

In post-menopausal women, movement regulates estrogen levels, helping manage weight, sleep, and mood swings. It's not about being a fitness fanatic—it's about choosing vitality.

Real-Life Inspiration:

Ernestine Shepherd: At 86, she's the world's oldest competitive female bodybuilder. She started exercising at 56 and proves it's never too late to reclaim your health.

Kiran Dembla: A mother and classical singer turned bodybuilder in her 40s, Kiran transformed her life through consistent workouts and now trains celebrities, motivating women across the country.

Saraswati's Story: At 64, Saraswati from Pune began simple stretching and walking after her granddaughter encouraged her. In just 3 months, her blood sugar stabilized, and her smile returned. "I feel 10 years younger," she says.

2: Simple At-Home Exercises for Strength, Flexibility & Balance

You don't need fancy equipment. Your home can be your personal fitness studio.

Strength Training (2–3 times a week)

- Wall push-ups
- Chair squats
- Arm curls with water bottles
- Step-ups using stairs
- Resistance band pulls

Strength training is vital to maintain muscle mass, support joints, and increase metabolism. Just 15 minutes can make a difference.

Flexibility (Daily)

- Cat-Cow stretch
- Shoulder rolls
- Gentle seated twists
- Neck tilts
- Standing forward bends

Flexibility improves range of motion, making daily activities easier—from bending to pick up groceries to getting up from the floor.

Balance Exercises

- Standing on one leg (with support)
- Heel-to-toe walk
- Side leg raises
- Clock reach (imagine reaching to different times around you)
- Tai Chi-inspired movements

Balance work helps reduce the risk of falls, which is crucial for women in their 50s and beyond.

Tip: *Always warm up, wear comfortable clothes, and stay hydrated.*

Story: Meera's Morning Movement

At 58, Meera began her day with 10 minutes of stretches. Her chronic back pain reduced, her mobility improved, and she felt more alive than she had in years.

Bonus Tip: *Use simple tools like a towel for resistance stretches or a sturdy chair for support during standing exercises.*

3: How to Build an Enjoyable Workout Routine That Fits Your Lifestyle

The secret to sticking with fitness? Joy.

Make It Enjoyable:

- ✓ Play your favorite music and dance
- ✓ Join a virtual class with friends
- ✓ Walk with your spouse or neighbor
- ✓ Create themed workout days (Yoga Monday, Dance Wednesday)

Keep It Realistic:

- ✓ Start with 10–15 minutes a day
- ✓ Pick the best time (morning or post-tea)

✓ Alternate between types of workouts

Joyful movement releases stress and builds emotional resilience. Pair your workout with things you love: music, nature, laughter, or company.

Story: Priya's Dance Workout

Priya, 54, found joy in Bollywood dancing. Her living room became her studio. In 6 months, she shed inches, boosted her energy, and rediscovered her passion.

Weekly Routine Sample:

Monday: Morning yoga (15 min)

Tuesday: Evening walk (20 min)

Wednesday: Dance video workout (15 min)

Thursday: Chair strength training (15 min)

Friday: Restorative stretching (10 min)

Saturday: Outdoor activity (gardening, park walk)

Sunday: Rest or deep breathing with music

Role of Consistency: Your Magic Key to Transformation

"Consistency is the key to mastery. Do something daily, and results are inevitable."

Consistency provides emotional stability in a changing world. It makes exercise a habit, not a chore.

To Be Super Consistent:

- ✓ Set realistic, clear goals (10 min walk daily)
- ✓ Create a schedule and stick to it
- ✓ Start small and increase gradually
- ✓ Mix up routines: walk, yoga, dance
- ✓ Have accountability buddies (friends/family)
- ✓ Track your progress (wall calendar or app)
- ✓ Prepare in advance (clothes, water, mat)
- ✓ Make a "power spot" at home for workouts
- ✓ Reward yourself (e.g., after 10 sessions, treat yourself)

Mini Reward Ideas:

- Buy a new scarf after 2 weeks of consistency
- Treat yourself to herbal tea or a pedicure

"When you're consistent, your body begins to trust you—and that's when real change begins."

4: Overcoming Common Fitness Challenges (Joint Pain, Stiffness, Fatigue)

1. Joint Pain & Stiffness:

1. Use hot compress or warm baths
2. Try water therapy or low-impact yoga
3. Focus on mobility routines
4. Include anti-inflammatory foods like turmeric, ginger

Bonus Tip: *Aloe vera juice, calcium-rich foods, and omega-3 supplements can support joint health.*

2. Low Energy:

1. Light meal before workout
2. Choose time with natural energy (morning)
3. Don't overtrain. Start small.
4. Drink enough water throughout the day

Try This: *Lemon water with a pinch of pink salt before a workout to boost hydration.*

3. Lack of Motivation:

1. Set simple goals: 20 walks in a month
2. Track your progress with a journal or app
3. Celebrate your wins
4. Join a support group

Story: Asha's Comeback

At 61, Asha struggled with arthritis. Chair yoga became her anchor. Slowly, she reduced pain, built stamina, and started a wellness circle in her apartment.

Incorporating Movement into Everyday Life

You don't need a formal workout to stay active.

Ideas to Stay Moving Throughout the Day:

- ✓ Take short walks every 2 hours
- ✓ Use stairs instead of elevators
- ✓ Practice desk stretches while sitting
- ✓ Stand while folding laundry or watching TV
- ✓ Dance breaks: 5-minute joy sessions
- ✓ Gardening, sweeping, or light housework
- ✓ Walk with pets or grandchildren
- ✓ Download fitness apps like Fittr or MyFitnessPal

New Additions:

Use a step tracker for friendly competition with family

Host "wellness tea time" with neighbors where everyone stretches and sips

Story: Rekha's Rhythms

At 60, Rekha began dancing to old Hindi songs while cooking. Her daughter gifted her ankle bells. Today, it's her daily cardio with joy!

Real Women, Real Wins

Maria, 56: From 5-minute balcony strolls to 3 km daily walks.

Lisa, 59: Overcame post-surgery fatigue through slow pranayama and regained lung strength.

Lakshmi, 62: Began indoor yoga and later trained as a yoga instructor for seniors.

Nirmala, 65: Switched to walking meditation and lost 5 kgs over 8 months.

Overcoming Barriers to Physical Activity

Set a vision: What do you want to achieve? More energy? Better mood?

Create a schedule: Create a realistic schedule that works with your day.

Make it social: Invite friends or join a local wellness group.

Incorporate variety: Alternate between walking, dancing, games.

Adapt: Short workouts when traveling, indoor walks during monsoon.

Invest in comfort: Shoes, soft mats, breathable clothes.

Handle discomfort: Modify moves, rest when needed.

Use technology: YouTube, fitness apps, WhatsApp wellness groups.

Celebrate: Track progress and reward milestones.

"Movement isn't a task—it's a gift to yourself."

Key Takeaways

- ✓ Movement is medicine: Begin with 10 minutes daily
- ✓ Age is not a barrier—it's a reason to start
- ✓ Make it fun, varied, and joyful
- ✓ Be consistent: habits build resilience
- ✓ Celebrate effort over perfection

"Your body will thank you for every move you make."

Closing Message: Keep Moving, Keep Glowing

Fitness isn't about looking a certain way—it's about feeling alive, empowered, and radiant. Whether you stretch on your mat, walk in your lane, or dance in your kitchen, your body and spirit will respond with joy.

You are not too old. You are perfectly poised to blossom. Move with grace. Live with fire.

"Move not to lose weight, but to gain life."

Your Personal Movement Action Plan

✓ Choose a consistent time daily (morning/evening)

✓ Keep workout clothes and mat ready

✓ Use a playlist of your favorite energizing songs

✓ Pick 3 core movements for the day (walk, stretch, strength)

✓ Track your days and reward your streaks

✓ Share your wins with a friend or group

✓ Add joyful movement: dance, play, garden

✓ Make fitness your celebration, not obligation

"Let your movement be your love letter to the life you want."

■ ■ ■

Chapter 3: Fueling Your Fabulous – Nutrition for Energy and Vitality

"Let food be thy medicine and medicine be thy food."
– Hippocrates

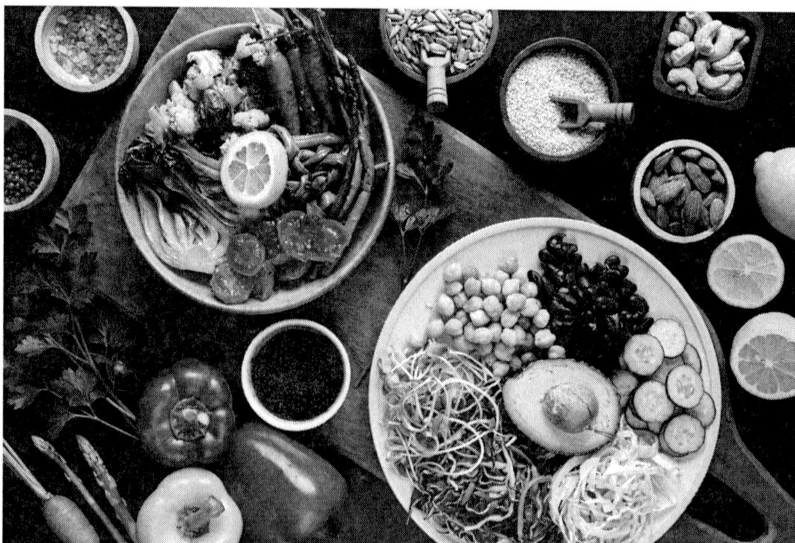

The Power of Food – More Than Just Fuel

I was in my early forties when I realized how deeply my food choices influenced my energy, mood, and overall vitality. For years, I had been juggling the home, raising children, managing guests, and putting everyone else's needs ahead of mine. Meals were hurried, often skipped, or filled with tea and processed snacks.

One evening, after an especially exhausting day, I

watched my mother sitting peacefully at the dinner table. Her skin glowed. She was smiling and eating slowly, enjoying every bite.

"Ma, how do you always have so much energy?" I asked.

She looked up and said gently, "I listen to my body. I eat what nourishes me, not just what fills me. If you treat food as your medicine, you'll never feel exhausted."

That night, I made a promise to myself. I would stop eating on autopilot. I would be mindful. I would nourish, not just consume. I began by adding colorful veggies to my plate, replacing sugary tea with warm lemon water, and including a protein source in every meal. I made it a point to sit down while eating, chew properly, and express gratitude for my food.

These small shifts created magic. I felt lighter, more energetic, and more in tune with my body. The fog lifted. I realized that mindful, wholesome eating isn't about diets. It's a way of loving yourself.

Now, let's walk together into this world of nourishment and rediscover the joy of food.

1: Foods that Support Strong Bones, Glowing Skin, and a Sharp Mind

---

"The food you eat can be either the safest and most powerful form of medicine or the slowest form of poison." – Ann Wigmore

---

After 50, the body naturally changes, making it even more important to choose food that heals, strengthens, and energizes.

Key Changes in the Body

- Slower metabolism – Requires nutrient-dense foods over calorie-rich junk
- Muscle loss (Sarcopenia) – Needs more protein for preservation
- Hormonal changes – Affect appetite, mood, and digestion
- Bone loss – Demands calcium and Vitamin D
- Decreased hydration – Need to drink more water consciously

"Your kitchen is your wellness pharmacy. Choose wisely."

Protein for Strength

Sources: Moong dal, chana, paneer, curd, tofu, sprouts, eggs, fish, chicken

Quick Recipe – Moong Dal Chilla: Soak 1 cup moong dal, grind with green chili, ginger & cumin. Add chopped onions. Cook like dosa. Serve with mint chutney

Pro Tip: *Begin your day with protein for sustained energy.*

Calcium and Vitamin D for Bone Strength

Sources: Milk, curd, paneer, ragi, sesame seeds, almonds, spinach, methi

Recipe– Ragi Porridge: Mix 2 tbsp ragi flour with milk and jaggery. Add cardamom and cook until creamy. Add ghee.

Pro Tip: *Soak in early morning sunlight for 15 minutes daily for natural Vitamin D.*

Healthy Fats for Brain & Skin Health

Sources: Ghee (moderate), nuts, seeds, avocado, cold-pressed oils

Recipe – Masala Buttermilk: Blend curd, water, roasted cumin, salt, ginger, coriander.

Pro Tip: *A spoon of ghee improves absorption and joint health.*

Iron and B12 to Fight Fatigue

Sources: Greens, lentils, jaggery, bajra, ragi, dry fruits, dairy, eggs

Recipe – Dry Fruit Ladoos: Roast almonds, dates, figs, walnuts. Add grated jaggery and ghee. Roll into balls.

Pro Tip: *Pair iron with lemon juice for absorption.*

Additional Practical Tips:

1. Add turmeric and black pepper in dals and curries for anti-inflammatory benefits.
2. Sprinkle flax seeds in your chapati dough or salad.

3. Use steel or clay cookware to avoid toxins and retain nutrients.

Real-Life Story – Shanta's Skin Glow Journey:

Shanta, a 57-year-old teacher, struggled with dull skin. Her granddaughter suggested almonds soaked overnight, green smoothies, and a flaxseed spoon daily. Within months, her skin glowed, and confidence grew.

2: The Importance of Hydration and Gut Health

As women enter their 50s and beyond, their bodies undergo significant hormonal and physiological changes. Staying at home, with often less structured routines and physical activity, can sometimes cause important aspects of wellness—like hydration and gut health—to be overlooked. However, these two simple yet powerful elements play a crucial role in maintaining energy, immunity, digestion, skin glow, and even emotional balance.

Why Hydration MattersMore After 50

Water is the foundation of life. Yet, as we age, our sense of thirst naturally diminishes, which means you may not feel thirsty even when your body desperately needs fluids. Dehydration is more common in older adults and can lead to fatigue, headaches, dry skin, dizziness, and even constipation.

For women over 50, adequate hydration helps:

1. Lubricate joints and reduce stiffness
2. Maintain skin elasticity and reduce the appearance of wrinkles

3. Regulate body temperature, especially during hot flashes or menopausal symptoms
4. Flush toxinsfrom the body and support kidney function
5. Improve digestion and prevent constipation

Practical Tips:

- ✓ Start your day with a glass of warm water with lemon.
- ✓ Sip herbal teas (like tulsi or ginger) throughout the day.
- ✓ Keep a water bottle nearby—even during indoor tasks.
- ✓ Eat water-rich foods like cucumbers, oranges, watermelon, and soups.
- ✓ Set reminders if you often forget to drink.
- ✓ Aim for at least 8–10 glasses of water daily, adjusting for climate and activity levels.

Gut Health: Your Second Brain

Did you know that nearly 70% of your immune system resides in your gut? Or that your gut produces 90% of the body's serotonin, the hormone that regulates mood?

A healthy gut means better digestion, stronger immunity, clearer thinking, and a more stable mood. But many women over 50 face digestive issues—bloating, acid reflux, irregular bowels—due to reduced metabolism, stress, or changes in hormone levels.

A strong gut can help you:

1. Absorb nutrients better from the food you eat
2. Reduce inflammation and chronic fatigue
3. Improve your mood and mental clarity
4. Enhance your immune response to infections

Simple Ways to Improve Gut Health:

✓ Add fiber-rich foods: whole grains, lentils, leafy greens, fruits like papaya and guava

✓ Eat fermented foods like curd, idli, dosa, kanji, or homemade pickle (in moderation)

✓ Take probiotics naturally (curd, buttermilk) or as supplements if advised

✓ Avoid overuse of antibiotics and processed foods

✓ Chew your food slowly and mindfully to aid digestion

Fiber for Digestive Health

Sources: Oats, millets, brown rice, papaya, apple, pumpkin, bhindi, chia, flax seeds

Recipe – Chia Pudding: Soak 2 tbsp chia seeds in almond milk overnight. Add honey, walnuts, pomegranate.

Pro Tip: *Soak flax/ chia in warm water to aid digestion.*

Morning Hydration Rituals:

Start with warm lemon water, jeera/ajwain water, or soaked methi seeds.

Probiotic Foods for Gut Health:

Curd, buttermilk, fermented rice, kanji, homemade pickles

Extra Tips:

1. Add a pinch of hing (asafoetida) in dal for better digestion.
2. Sip warm fennel tea after meals to reduce bloating.
3. Avoid drinking water right after meals—wait 30 minutes.

Uma's Gut Revival: Uma, 61, often felt bloated. She began including probiotic curd and warm lemon water. Within weeks, her energy returned, and digestion improved.

"Your gut is your second brain—feed it well and feel the difference."

Final Thought:

Hydration and gut health may seem like small parts of the wellness puzzle, but they are powerful. By drinking enough water and caring for your digestive system, you support every other system in your body—from your brain to your bones. It's not about a complete overhaul—it's about honoring your body with the basics. **Sip. Chew. Nourish. Glow.**

3. Meal Planning and Easy, Nutritious Recipes

The Ideal Plate: 50% vegetables, 25% protein, 25% whole grains, 1 tsp healthy fat

Sample Day Plan:

Morning: Lemon water

Breakfast: Moong chilla + fruit

Mid-morning: Buttermilk + almonds

Lunch: Brown rice + dal + sabzi + curd

Evening: Roasted chana or fruit salad

Dinner: Roti + palak paneer + pumpkin sabzi

Bedtime: Haldi milk or chamomile tea

Smart Prep Tips:

Plan a weekly menu—simplifies shopping and reduces waste.

Store cooked dal and veggies for 2 days in advance.

Use a chalkboard or sticky note in your kitchen for tracking.

Easy Recipe – Immunity Soup: Boil carrots, tomatoes, beetroot, garlic, and ginger. Blend. Add pepper and lemon.

Real-Life Story – Latha's 30-Minute Routine: Latha, 55, cared for her in-laws. She prepped weekly veggies, stored pre-soaked lentils, and followed a "Tuesday to Saturday" menu plan. Her energy soared.

4. Managing Cravings and Maintaining a Balanced Diet

Mindful Eating Practices:

✓ Avoid screens while eating

✓ Sit down and eat slowly

✓ Use clay or brass utensils

✓ Light a diya before meals

✓ Practice gratitude

Smart Tips to Beat Cravings:

Sweet: Dates with almonds, jaggery chikki

Salty: Roasted peanuts, baked khakra

Spicy: Masala buttermilk or lemon pickle with sprouts

Right Eating Habits:

✓ Eat every 3-4 hours

✓ Balance all 5 food groups

✓ Hydrate with herbal teas

✓ Avoid white sugar, processed food

Real-Life Story – Rekha's Sugar Shift:

Rekha, 59, replaced biscuits with fruit and cinnamon. She switched to dry fruit laddoos and noticed less fatigue.

"Balanced eating is not about discipline —it's about self-respect."

Consistency is Key:

Don't aim for perfection. Keep showing up.

Celebrate small wins—7 days of mindful eating = treat yourself to a book or spa.

Real-Life Inspiration – Nirmala's Rituals:

Nirmala, a retired principal, lived alone. She set a table, played soft music, and lit a lamp before meals. Her mood improved, and she began to savor every bite.

Inspiring Indian Women Who Prioritize Wellness

Anshu Jamsenpa – The first Indian woman to summit Everest twice in five days. Her secret: a clean Himalayan diet.

Dinaz Vervatwala – A fitness coach in her 50s, known for her balanced diet and focus on women's wellness.

Shobha, 64 – Homemaker-turned-YouTuber sharing nutritious recipes that inspire thousands of women post-50.

Conclusion: Your Health, Your Choice

"When you nourish your body,
you nourish your spirit."

Food is your fuel, your friend, and your foundation. As a woman over 50, your body is wise. Now, fuel it with kindness, consistency, and care.

Eat with joy. Cook with love. Live with vitality.

Fabulous Nutrition Action Plan

✓ Start with lemon or methi water

✓ Eat 3 meals + 2 snacks

✓ Include one leafy green daily

✓ Try 2 new recipes weekly

✓ Hydrate well – 8-10 glasses

✓ Practice gratitude before meals

✓ Avoid screens while eating

✓ Swap processed food for fresh

"Let your plate be a celebration of your strength and joy."

■ ■ ■

Chapter 4: Stress Less, Live More – Mastering Emotional Wellness

"It's not stress that kills us, it is our reaction to it." — Hans Selye

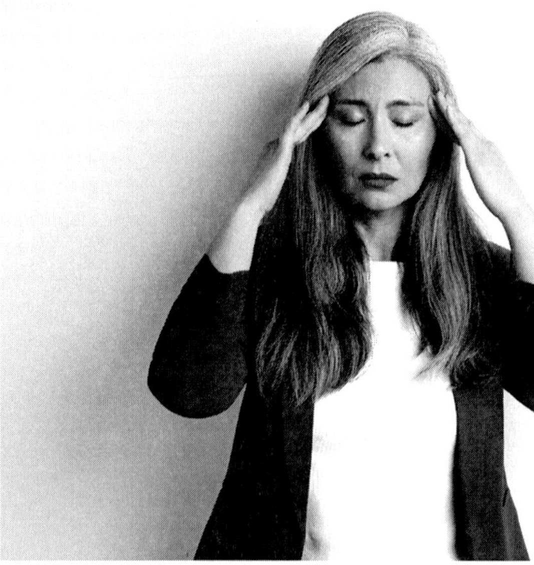

Introduction: A Gentle Revolution Within

Stress doesn't announce itself with fanfare. It creeps in slowly—in the fatigue behind our smiles, the weight in our shoulders, the moments we forget to breathe. For women over 50, especially those staying at home, emotional wellness often takes a backseat. We're taught to care for others, to give endlessly. But peace, like joy, begins within.

This chapter is an invitation to reclaim your calm, to rewrite the rhythm of your day with grace, stillness, and strength. Through stories, techniques, and rituals, let's discover how to stress less and live more—authentically, joyfully, and fully.

1. Understanding Stress and Its Impact on Your Body and Mind

The day my daughter gave birth was one of the happiest in my life. Our home was bursting with love. My elder daughter, son-in-law, and grandchildren were all under one roof. Laughter echoed in every corner, and a warm sense of celebration filled the air.

But beneath that joy, I felt something different—an ache. From dawn till night, I cooked, cleaned, and cradled little ones. I greeted everyone with a smile, but inside, I was drained. Sleep was elusive, and by evening, I felt like I was running on empty.

The next morning, I shared this with a close friend whose energy always amazed me. Her calm face, gentle voice, and glowing skin were a mystery I now wanted to understand.

She smiled and said, "I make stress relief a priority."

She shared her simple, life-changing morning rituals:

1. 5 minutes of deep breathing
2. A warm glass of water with lemon
3. Stretching to soft instrumental music
4. Sipping tea mindfully without screens

5. Reading a positive affirmation aloud

Inspired, I tried her routine the next day. That tiny pocket of peace became my sacred start. I slowly felt lighter, more grounded, and more present.

I danced with my grandchildren. I took power naps without guilt. I journaled. And most of all, I smiled at myself in the mirror—a smile of self-recognition.

A Garden of Peace – My Friend Sujatha's Story

While I found peace in mindful living, my friend Sujatha discovered hers in the soil.

After retiring from her teaching job, Sujatha felt lost. Her days felt hollow. That's when she stepped onto her small terrace and noticed the lonely pots.

She began with coriander and tulsi. Then came tomatoes, okra, and brinjal. Every morning, Sujatha spent an hour watering, pruning, and talking to her plants. She played bhajans softly and whispered gratitude to every blooming flower.

In her words:

> *"Gardening gave my days meaning. Watching something grow under your care is therapy."*

Today, Sujatha's green haven not only feeds her body but heals her soul. Neighbors visit her garden for advice—and inspiration.

Why Stress Management Matters for Women Over 50

Stress isn't just emotional. For women over 50, it has

profound physical and mental consequences.

Key Challenges Include:

- Hormonal Changes – Menopause brings mood swings, hot flashes, and sleep issues.
- Physical Strain – Joint pain, fatigue, and sluggishness amplify with unmanaged stress.
- Emotional Weight – Empty nests, caregiving roles, and shifting identities weigh heavily.
- Chronic stress increases cortisol, accelerates aging, weakens immunity, and dulls our inner glow.

"Managing stress is not optional. It is essential self-care."

Understanding Stress and Its Hidden Impact

Stress is a survival mechanism. But when it stays too long, it harms more than it helps.

Physical Symptoms:

- Constant fatigue and tension headaches
- Indigestion, acidity, and weight gain
- Brain fog and memory lapses

Emotional Effects:

- Mood swings, irritability, and anxiety
- Depression or feeling "empty"

Real-Life Insight: Rekha's Realization

Rekha, a retired teacher, loved staying active. But fatigue and insomnia plagued her. A check-up revealed high cortisol. Through journaling, slow yoga, and mindful breathing, she reclaimed her energy. She now leads a wellness WhatsApp group for seniors.

2. Practical Relaxation Techniques (Breathing Exercises, Meditation, Journaling)

Deep Breathing – The 4-7-8 Method

- Inhale through the nose for 4 seconds
- Hold for 7 seconds
- Exhale through the mouth for 8 seconds
- Repeat 4-6 times daily

Gentle Exercise & Yoga

- Child's Pose – Relaxes the spine
- Legs-Up-the-Wall – Relieves tension
- 10-minute sunrise stretch – Boosts circulation

Meditation & Visualization

- Use apps like Insight Timer, Sattva, or Calm
- Visualize a peaceful scene: a river, temple, or garden

Journaling

- Write 3 things you're grateful for each night
- Let out your thoughts like a conversation with your heart

Music & Movement

- Dance while cooking
- Play nostalgic songs or bhajans

3. How to Set Boundaries and Prioritize Self-Care

"You can't pour from an empty cup."

For generations, women have been celebrated as nurturers—the ones who hold families together with love, attention, and care. While this role is honorable, it often comes at the cost of their own well-being. After 50, when the body and mind require more gentleness and restoration, self-neglect can quietly take a toll. Setting boundaries is not selfish—it is essential. And self-care is not an indulgence—it is a necessity for physical, mental, and emotional balance.

How to Set Healthy Boundaries:

Most women over 50 have spent decades saying "yes"—to family, work, neighbors, and social obligations. But the truth is, saying "yes" to everything often means saying "no" to yourself. Setting boundaries begins with recognizing your limits and honoring them.

Make a list of draining tasks and delegate

Identify tasks that exhaust you—be it endless WhatsApp groups, overcommitting to social gatherings, or handling chores others can do. Delegate household responsibilities to family members. Involve your children or spouse in meal planning, errands, or tech issues. Sharing the load lightens your mind and strengthens bonds.

Say "no" without guilt

"No" is a full sentence. You don't owe anyone an elaborate excuse for preserving your energy. Declining an event or favor allows space for things that align with your wellness. Every time you say "yes" to something that drains you, you're saying "no" to your own peace. Flip the script—yes to self means no to overwhelm.

Block 'me-time' like an important appointment

Add your self-time to your calendar—just like doctor appointments or family events. Whether it's 15 minutes of silence in the morning or a creative hour in the evening, protect it. Treat this time with respect and consistency. The more you honor it, the more others will too.

Self-Care Practices that Replenish:

Self-care doesn't always mean elaborate spa days. Often, it's in the small, consistent rituals that soothe the soul and recharge the spirit.

Morning tea alone, gazing out the window

Let the first few minutes of the day belong to you. Sip your tea slowly. Watch the sunrise. Feel the breeze. Let your thoughts wander without urgency. These quiet moments set a peaceful tone for the day.

An evening ritual—music, light, and silence

Create a calming environment as the day winds down. Soft instrumental music, a candle or dim lamp, and a few minutes of silence can help transition from "doing" to simply "being." Reflect. Breathe. Let go of the day's heaviness.

Hobbies like knitting, mandala art, or puzzles

Creative hobbies offer meditative focus and joy. Whether it's painting, gardening, or solving puzzles, engaging your hands calms your mind. These activities serve as gentle therapy—no screens, no pressure, just presence.

Example: Priya's Shift

Priya, 54, was the classic giver—always available, always saying "yes." Eventually, burnout caught up. One day, she picked up her daughter's unused paint set and began painting quietly in the corner of her bedroom. That 30-minute ritual became her sanctuary. In just weeks, her family noticed her lighter mood, her glow. That small act restored her calm and, more importantly, her sense of self-worth.

How to Set Healthy Boundaries:

- Make a list of draining tasks and delegate
- Say "no" without guilt—yes to self means no to overwhelm
- Block "me-time" like an important appointment

Self-Care Practices:

- Morning tea alone, gazing out the window
- An evening ritual—music, light, and silence
- Hobbies like knitting, mandala art, or puzzle

4. Cultivating Joy Through Hobbies and Passions

Joy heals. Passion anchors us.

Why It Matters:

- Releases dopamine, the joy hormone
- Enhances creativity and mindfulness
- Connects us to our purpose

Joyful Activities to Try:

- Gardening, embroidery, or painting
- Singing bhajans or learning an instrument
- Reading spiritual or historical novels
- Teaching a skill online or mentoring youth

Suman's Second Spring

At 56, Suman reignited her passion for painting. She opened an Instagram page, shared her art, and even sold a few pieces. Her joy became her fuel.

Bonus Section: Building Resilience for Long-Term Wellness

1. Mindset Shift

- Reframe: Every challenge is a redirection
- Speak kindly to yourself daily

2. Support Systems

- Lean on trusted friends
- Join women's wellness or gratitude circles

3. Flexibility

- Let go of rigidity
- Adapt your routines with grace

4. Gratitude Practice

- Write 3 good things each night
- Share one thank-you message weekly

5. Purpose-Driven Living

- Start a balcony herb garden
- Record your life stories for your grandchildren
- Support a local NGO

Inspiration: Kiran Mazumdar-Shaw

India's pioneering biotech entrepreneur faced immense stress in a male-dominated field. But with calm, courage, and community support, she built an empire that heals.

Final Thoughts – Your Joyful Life Begins Now

Stress is real, but so is your ability to rise.

Emotional wellness is a gift you give yourself daily—in pauses, in peace, in play. From mindful rituals to joyful movements, this is your time to soften the edges and sparkle from within.

"You owe yourself the love you so freely give to others."

Your Action Plan – *Tick Off Your Daily Joy Rituals!*

- Morning breathing + gratitude journaling
- 10-minute walk or gentle yoga
- A nourishing breakfast with music
- One creative or joyful hobby
- A phone call with a friend
- 30 minutes of screen-free rest before bed

"Stress less, live more, love yourself first —and the rest will follow."

■ ■ ■

Chapter 5: Beauty from the Inside Out – Radiate Confidence at Any Age

"Beauty begins the moment you decide to be yourself." – Coco Chanel

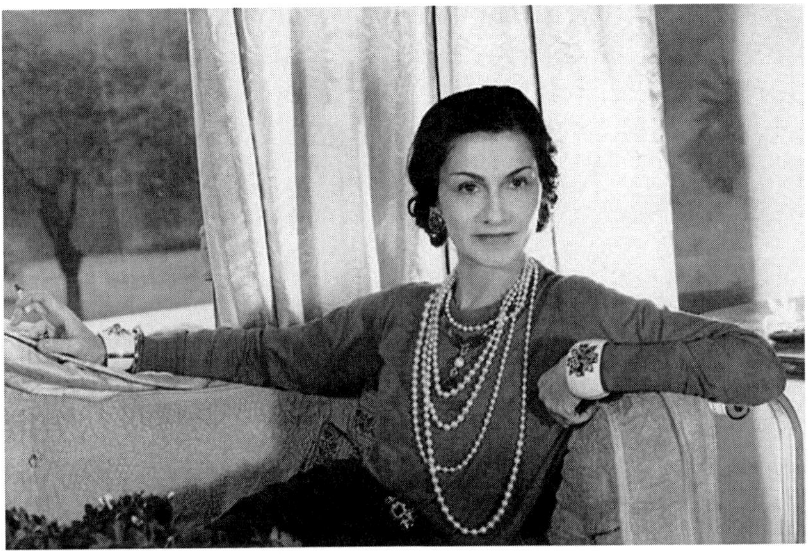

The Timeless Glow of Confidence

They say beauty is in the eye of the beholder—but what if the most important beholder is you?

Confidence, self-care, and a touch of radiance can make any woman shine at any age. You don't need expensive products or cosmetic fixes. True beauty comes from how you treat yourself, how you see yourself, and how you honor your essence.

Beauty at 50 and beyond is not about chasing youth; it is about embracing your story, nurturing your spirit, and walking through life with vibrancy. This chapter is your invitation to reconnect with your inner light and radiate beauty that is timeless.

A Personal Story – A House of Love and a Mirror of Realization

During the summer, we visited my mother's place with the children for a few weeks. It was a house full of love, laughter, noise, and endless joy. We had our cousins, relatives, little ones running around with nonstop chatter, meals that brought everyone together, and late-night laughs. I enjoyed every moment, surrounded by the warmth of family.

But one quiet afternoon, I stepped into the bedroom for a few minutes of rest. Everyone else was busy chatting in the living room. As I sat on the bed, I caught a glimpse of myself in the mirror. For the first time in weeks, I looked at myself—not just glanced, but really looked. My skin looked dull, my hair messy, and my face carried visible fatigue.

That moment was a revelation. I realized I had been so caught up in serving, feeding, entertaining, and organizing that I had completely ignored myself. My daily skincare had been forgotten, I wore the same comfortable clothes each day without much thought, and I had not even smiled at my reflection.

I remembered my mother's precious advice:

- Focus on yourself each day, even in the midst of service.
- Eat nourishing food and savor it with gratitude.

- Sleep peacefully, letting go of the day with a smile.
- Spend a few minutes in silence to center your spirit.
- Keep moving - walk, stretch, dance.
- Smile often, for it lights you up within.
- Engage joyfully with others, share laughter.
- Thank your body daily for carrying you with strength.
- Think positively, because what you believe, you attract.

Her words echoed like a warm hug.

That day, I took a long, soothing shower, wore a fresh kurta, applied moisturizer, lined my eyes softly, and adorned a little bindi. When I smiled into the mirror, the reflection smiled back—alive, radiant, present.

It was not about impressing others. It was about respecting myself. That evening, my daughter whispered, "Amma, you look so beautiful today." That single comment filled my heart with immense warmth.

This journey taught me that true beauty blooms from self-love, mindfulness, and daily care.

1. Skincare Routines for Mature Skin

"Invest in your skin. It is going to represent you for a very long time."

With time, our skin naturally changes, but with nurturing, it can glow with health and pride.

Essential Skincare for Women 50+:

Gentle Cleansing: Choose hydrating cream- or oil-based cleansers to maintain natural oils.

Hydrating Toner: Pure rose water or hyaluronic acid toners restore freshness.

Nourishing Serums: Vitamin C serums brighten skin; retinol boosts collagen gently.

Daily Moisturizer: Look for ceramides and peptides for elasticity and protection.

Sunscreen Always: SPF 30+ every single day—indoors and outdoors.

Mini Ritual: Warm a few drops of almond oil and massage your face at night with gratitude—thank each feature that smiles, speaks, and expresses.

Rekha's Glow-Up: At 58, Rekha switched to simple products and consistency. Within months, her skin looked hydrated, lively, and she radiated confidence—barefaced and beautiful.

Motivating Tip: *Glow comes from care, not layers of makeup. Choose nourishment over camouflage.*

2. The Role of Sleep in Beauty and Aging Gracefully

"Sleep is the best meditation." – Dalai Lama

Your body's repair workshop is active during sleep. Missing rest steals your radiance.

Restorative Sleep Tips:

Consistent Schedule: Sleep and rise at the same times daily.

Evening Calm: Herbal tea, soft lighting, and light stretches.

Silk Pillowcases: Reduce skin creases and hair breakage.

No Screens Zone: Avoid screens an hour before sleep.

Meena's Story: Struggling with insomnia, Meena began a nightly ritual—chamomile tea, lavender oil massage, and gratitude journaling. Her inner glow returned, and she looked visibly fresher and joyful.

Motivating Tip: *Sleep isn't a luxury—it's the foundation of beauty and wellness.*

3. Embracing Natural Beauty and Self-Expression

"Be your own kind of beautiful."

Authenticity is the most stunning accessory.

Celebrate Your Natural Beauty:

Colorful Plates: Antioxidant-rich foods heal skin from inside.

Hydration Habit: Sip water often—add cucumber, mint, or lemon.

Enhance, Don't Mask: Tinted moisturizer, kohl, and lip tints bring softness.

The Power of a Smile: Light up rooms with your presence.

Kavita's Confidence Shift: Kavita, 55, embraced her silver hair with grace. She wore colorful scarves, bold lipstick, and a magnetic smile—drawing admiration and sparking conversations.

Motivating Tip: *When you honor your authentic beauty, the world reflects it back with love.*

4. Fashion and Styling Tips to Feel Confident at Home and Beyond

---

"Style is a way to say who you are without having to speak."

Self-expression through style uplifts mood and spirit.

Wardrobe Essentials for Radiant Women:

Soft Cotton Kurtis and Flowy Tunics: Breathable and elegant.

Comfortable Palazzos, Sarees, or Leggings: Ease of movement.

Joyful Footwear: Pretty yet practical sandals.

Charming Accessories: Bright earrings, delicate scarves, silver bangles.

Good Innerwear: Supportive, comfortable, and uplifting.

Aditi's Transformation: Aditi swapped old nighties for colorful kurtas, feeling vibrant and alive. Her renewed confidence inspired her to start teaching music classes online.

Aunty Rekha's Elegance: At 65, Aunty Rekha wore soft silk sarees with fresh jasmine flowers in her hair. Her smile, poise, and loving energy made her unforgettable—a true role model for generations.

Motivating Tip: *Dress for yourself, honor your body, and walk proudly—even if you're simply at home.*

Conclusion: Your Confidence Is Your Signature

"Your beauty should not be defined by your age, but by your energy."

Confidence is an inner glow that radiates beyond makeup or fashion. It shines through your kindness, your gratitude, your joyful movement, and your love for life.

Age is a beautiful privilege. Each wrinkle, each silver strand, each laugh line tells your story.

Honor your body. Nurture your spirit. Nourish your dreams.

Your Action Plan for Radiant Living:

- Begin each morning with self-love: skincare, affirmations, gratitude.
- Prioritize good sleep—your nightly rejuvenation.
- Hydrate, nourish, and celebrate your body.
- Move daily—stretch, walk, or dance.
- Embrace your natural beauty—inside and out.

- Smile generously—at yourself and at others.
- Choose vibrant colors, flowing fabrics, and joyful accessories.

"Next time you look in the mirror,
smile at the woman looking back
—she's fabulous.
Let her shine, unapologetically."

■ ■ ■

Chapter 6: Keeping the Mind Sharp – Cognitive Health and Lifelong Learning

"You are never too old to set another goal or to dream a new dream." – C.S. Lewis

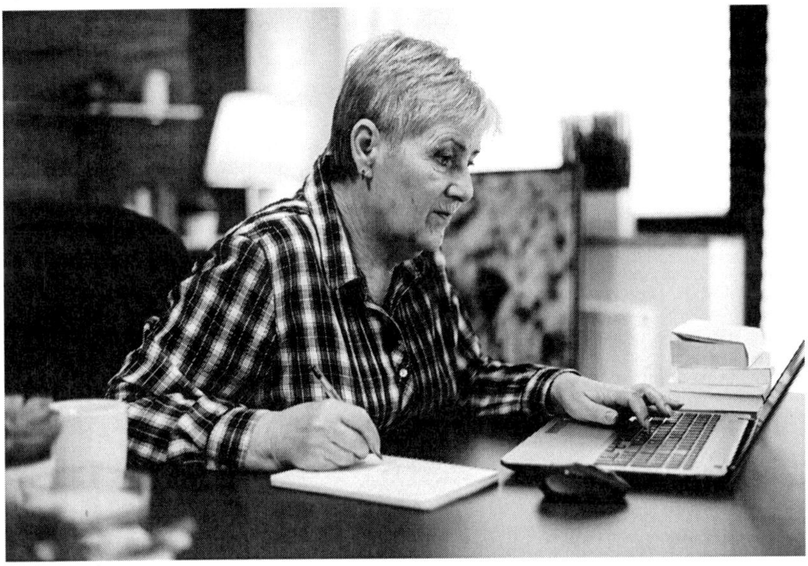

A New Beginning from Within

For years, I believed learning belonged in classrooms. But after I turned 50, I discovered a new kind of education—one that doesn't come with a certificate, but with joy, vitality, and mental freshness. It's a journey of lifelong curiosity, and it changed my life.

When my children moved away after their marriages, silence filled our home. The once-busy corners echoed with quiet, and I found myself slowly slipping into a monotonous routine. My energy dipped, my enthusiasm faded, and even my memory didn't feel as sharp. Days blurred into each other, and I questioned if this was how the rest of my life would feel.

Then came a spark of transformation—a dear friend introduced me to an online reading and brain-boosting community. She called it her "daily dose of joy." Intrigued, I joined. That single decision reignited my purpose.

The community offered beautifully curated modules: Memory Mastery, Speed Reading, Impromptu Speaking, and Creative Thinking. Each session was guided, interactive, and designed to keep our minds active and inspired.

Memory Mastery

This module introduced techniques like visualization, association, acronyms, and memory palaces. We practiced remembering names, grocery lists, book titles, and even shlokas. Within weeks, I could recall long passages and dates with surprising ease. It was empowering!

Speed Reading

We began with slow-paced reading and gradually increased speed without losing comprehension. Books like 'Think and Grow Rich' by Napoleon Hill and 'The 5 AM Club' by Robin Sharma weren't just reading material—they became my fuel. I learned to highlight, summarize, and apply concepts practically. This module revived my love for books.

Impromptu Speech

This was my favorite. We were asked to speak spontaneously on topics like "A dream I chased," or "My favorite childhood memory." At first, I was nervous. But soon, I began enjoying the flow of thoughts and words. Speaking up improved my confidence, vocabulary, and clarity.

These modules transformed my mornings. I now follow a 6-step morning ritual inspired by Hal Elrod's The Miracle Morning: Silence, Affirmations, Visualization, Exercise, Reading, and Scribing (journaling). This sacred hour boosts my clarity, creativity, and positivity.

Joining this circle of vibrant women brought back sparkle to my days. We learned together, laughed together, and grew together. I felt mentally sharper, emotionally grounded, and spiritually fulfilled.

1. How to Keep Your Brain Active and Engaged

"The mind is not a vessel to be filled, but a fire to be kindled." – Plutarch

A sharp mind is the strongest muscle we can train. Just like a body loses strength when unused, the mind too weakens without stimulation.

Daily Brain-Boosting Activities:

✓ Read articles, books, or poetry every day

✓ Solve puzzles: Sudoku, crosswords, jigsaw, or logic games

- ✓ Use brain-training apps like Lumosity, Peak, or Elevate
- ✓ Learn a new word daily and use it in conversation
- ✓ Join a quiz club or play mental games with your grandchildren

Story: Sarita, 62, from Kolkata

She enrolled in a digital painting course and used both visual and problem-solving skills. Her art was later featured in a senior's art exhibition.

2. The Benefits of Learning New Skills andTrying New Experiences

---

"Learning never exhausts the mind."
– Leonardo da Vinci

Midlife learning is a superpower. It enhances brain function and unlocks dormant creativity.

Why Learning After 50 is Powerful:

- Keeps neurons active, delaying cognitive decline
- Promotes happiness and combats depression
- Boosts decision-making, clarity, and reasoning
- Builds social interaction and confidence

Example: Lakshmi, 60

She started learning violin online and now performs at local community centers. She says, "I feel younger with every note I play."

Inspiring Women Icon: Sudha Murthy

Despite being a renowned author and philanthropist, she continues to explore new areas—from storytelling to social work. Her curiosity never retires.

3. Strategies for Improving Memory and Focus

Memory is a skill we can sharpen with consistent habits.

Proven Techniques:

✓ Chunking: Divide info into parts (e.g., break phone numbers into groups)

✓ Mnemonics: Use rhymes or acronyms to recall facts

✓ Association: Link new info to known visuals or events

✓ Teach Back: Explain what you learned to someone else

Brain-Healthy Habits:

✓ 7–8 hours of quality sleep

✓ 30 minutes of walking or gentle yoga daily

✓ Omega-3 rich diet (fish, flaxseed, walnuts)

✓ Meditation and breathwork (like 4-7-8 method)

4. The Power of Creativity and Curiosity

"Curiosity is the wick in the candle of learning."
– William Arthur Ward

Creativity isn't limited to artists. It's in how you cook, decorate, speak, and solve problems.

Ways to Spark Creativity:

✓ Write poems, blog posts, or family history

✓ Try DIY crafts or festive home decor

✓ Experiment in the kitchen with new recipes

✓ Start a gratitude jar or vision board

✓ Rearrange your furniture or redesign a room

Story: Manju, 65, Pune

Manju started writing haikus during the pandemic. Her short poems were later published in a local journal. "It helped me see beauty in small things," she shares.

Conclusion: Age is Just the Beginning

Midlife is not a slowing down—it's a beautiful awakening. You have the wisdom, time, and inner spark to reinvent your mental landscape.

✓ Keep learning: A curious brain is a youthful brain

✓ Stay social: Laughter and stories are the best stimulants

✓ Pursue joy: Learn for fun, not pressure

✓ Share your light: Teach, inspire, and uplift others

"Live as if you were to die tomorrow. Learn as if you were to live forever." – Mahatma Gandhi

---

You're not too old to begin—you're just getting started. Stay sharp, stay curious, and celebrate the fabulous learner within you.

■ ■ ■

Chapter 7: Staying Connected – Building a Supportive Community

"Connection is why we're here; it is what gives purpose and meaning to our lives." – Brené Brown

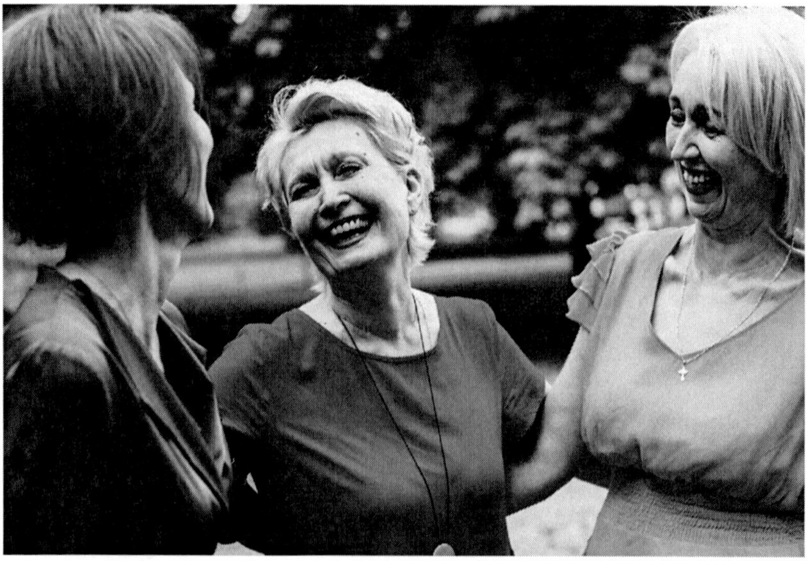

1. The Importance of Meaningful Relationships in Your 50s and Beyond

The Power of Connection: My Story of Transformation

As I shared earlier in this book, my journey into personal growth began when I stumbled upon an online reading and learning community. At the time, I was feeling directionless. With my children married and settled, the house echoed with a silence that once seemed peaceful, but now felt isolating. Days were consumed with routine—cooking, cleaning, and scrolling through social media without purpose.

One day, a friend invited me to join a virtual learning group that met every morning at 5:30 AM. At first, I hesitated. Would I fit in? Would I keep up?

But from the very first session, something awakened in me. We weren't just there to learn how to read faster or improve memory—we were building a circle of support, creativity, laughter, and empathy. That one hour every morning filled me with energy, clarity, and confidence that carried through the day.

I began to speak more confidently, explore new interests, and most importantly—I felt seen and valued. That group didn't just sharpen my mind; it opened my heart. It reminded me that meaningful connection is nourishment for the soul.

Why Staying Connected Matters After 50

At this stage of life, the world often expects us to take a backseat. But connection—true, meaningful connection—can be the very thing that rekindles our energy and self-worth.

- ✓ Emotional Upliftment – Even a small conversation can brighten a dull day
- ✓ Rekindled Energy – Anticipating a group activity or class boosts motivation
- ✓ Confidence Boost – Learning something new or sharing ideas builds pride
- ✓ Rediscovered Passions – Others can awaken forgotten dreams

✓ Deeper Friendships – Some online bonds grow even stronger than in-person ties

Real-Life Inspirations from Indian Women

Nalini (59, Pune) – Joined an online baking group and turned her hobby into a thriving home business.

Meena (64, Kochi) – Discovered a wellness WhatsApp group and developed a yoga and meditation habit.

Savitha (60, Delhi) – Became a virtual storyteller for children, winning hearts online.

Uma (62, Bengaluru) – Started writing poetry and published her first e-book.

Rekha (58, Nagpur) – Learned dance online, rediscovered joy, and performs at cultural events.

Shobha (65, Hyderabad) – Leads "Golden Circles," a WhatsApp group where women share daily gratitude and positivity.

These women show that it's never too late to begin again—and thrive.

How Meaningful Communities Bring Us Alive

When children leave the nest or careers wind down, it's easy to feel adrift. But meaningful communities bring new purpose, especially for women at home.

They can be:

- A learning group that boosts brain power
- A wellness circle for shared health goals
- A creative hub for art, music, or writing

- A support system for navigating menopause, grief, or transitions

Being part of something gives structure, joy, and a reason to wake up with purpose.

2. Ways to Stay Socially Engaged While Being at Home

How to Build Your Own Supportive Circle

Creating your own connection network can be simple and incredibly rewarding.

- ✓ Choose your joy – What do you love? Gardening, singing, reading?
- ✓ Start small – Invite a few friends or join a beginner's group
- ✓ Use tech tools – Zoom, WhatsApp, Facebook, Telegram
- ✓ Celebrate each other – Share wins, birthdays, or even small milestones
- ✓ Learn together – Watch TED Talks, take online courses, exchange books

***Tip**: Ask your grandchildren or younger relatives to teach you an app—it's a wonderful bonding activity too!*

Staying Socially Engaged from Home

You don't have to leave your home to stay connected. Here are some simple ways:

- ✓ Join hobby-based Facebook or WhatsApp groups
- ✓ Plan weekly virtual coffee chats or chai circles
- ✓ Start a neighborhood walking or book club
- ✓ Organize potluck dinners, poetry readings, or bhajan sessions
- ✓ Participate in virtual quizzes or craft workshops

Example: Suman, 61, organizes weekly Zoom chats with her sisters in different cities. These virtual catchups became their most cherished bonding time.

3. How to Use Technology to Connect with Loved Ones and Make New Friends

You don't have to be tech-savvy to enjoy the digital world.

- ✓ WhatsApp & Facebook – Family groups, sharing photos, wellness tips
- ✓ Zoom & Google Meet – Online learning, prayer groups, discussions
- ✓ Mobile Games – Play online Ludo, Scrabble, or chess with family
- ✓ Learning Platforms – Enroll in courses on Coursera, Udemy, Skillshare
- ✓ Virtual Events – Join book clubs, storytelling sessions, devotional gatherings

4. The Benefits of Volunteering and Giving Back

The Joy of Volunteering and Giving Back

Helping others boosts happiness and builds strong social bonds.

- ✓ Teach – Online or in-person, share cooking, sewing, or language skills
- ✓ Mentor – Guide younger women or students in career or life decisions
- ✓ Support Elders – Call senior citizens, help with tech or errands
- ✓ Community Work – Volunteer at NGOs, libraries, or health centers

Kavita's Story: A retired nurse, Kavita started mentoring young medical students through an NGO. "I feel younger and more alive when I share what I know," she says.

Activities for Physical, Social, and Mental Fitness

Here are simple ways to stay active and connected every day:

Physical:

- ✓ 15-minute morning walk with a friend
- ✓ Learn yoga or dance from YouTube
- ✓ Gardening or light housework as natural movement

Mental:

- ✓ Daily crossword or Sudoku
- ✓ Memory games with grandchildren
- ✓ Online workshops or writing circles

Social:

- ✓ Weekly group calls with friends
- ✓ Attend local women's meetups
- ✓ Start a digital scrapbook club with family

Emotional:

- ✓ Journaling about daily joys
- ✓ Gratitude group message every evening
- ✓ Share one new learning each week with a friend

Motivating Story: The Garden of Hope

Sujatha, 60, felt emotionally lost after retirement. On a whim, she began planting on her terrace. A few pots turned into a mini garden. Every morning, she watered her plants, listened to soft music, and journaled beside them.

Her garden became a space of healing and inspiration. Today, she shares photos and gardening tips in a WhatsApp group that has inspired dozens of women.

Your Connection Action Plan

- ✓ Join or create one online or offline community this month
- ✓ Host a chai chat with friends or neighbors
- ✓ Commit to a weekly joy circle—art, reading, prayer, or laughter
- ✓ Use one new app to connect with someone special
- ✓ Volunteer your time, wisdom, or talent once a week
- ✓ Start a gratitude chain message with five friends

Closing Reflections: Together, We Shine Brighter

Connection isn't a luxury—it's life-giving. Women, especially after 50, need connection not only for companionship, but for courage, joy, and purpose.

Your voice matters. Your experience inspires. Your kindness heals.

"In this circle, age doesn't define us —connection does."

So, reach out. Join in. Laugh loud. Give more. And receive the joy of being truly, beautifully connected.

■ ■ ■

Chapter 8: Overcoming Setbacks – Dealing with Health Challenges and Life Changes

"She stood in the storm, and when the wind did not blow her way, she adjusted her sails."
– Elizabeth Edwards

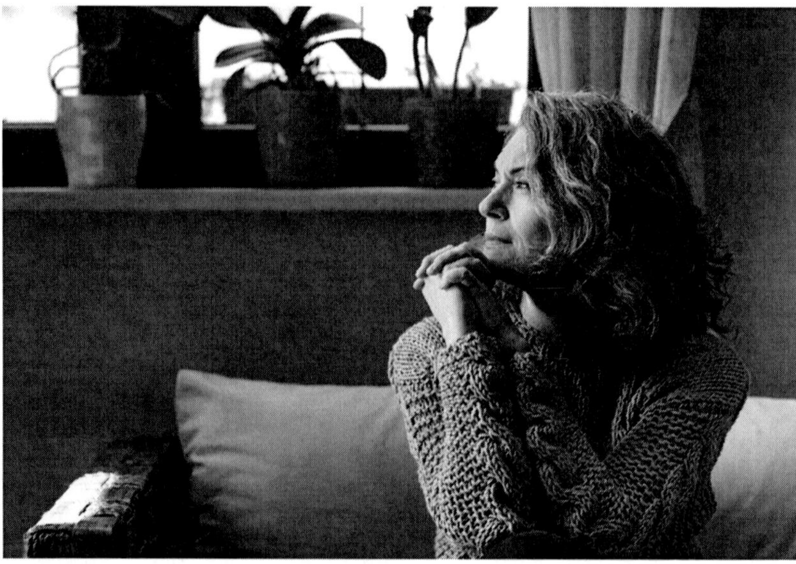

Strength in Adversity

Life after 50 is a vibrant yet delicate phase—filled with wisdom, transitions, and opportunities to rediscover oneself. Yet, it can also be marked by emotional challenges, physical changes, and personal losses. Menopause, retirement, loneliness, or health issues may seem like insurmountable obstacles.

But this chapter isn't about defeat—it's about rising, even stronger.

I still remember one quiet afternoon during my menopause phase. My mind felt clouded, my body fatigued. I had just finished cleaning up after a family gathering, and as I sat with a warm cup of ginger tea, I whispered to myself, "I need to do something for me."

That whisper became a turning point.

I began with five minutes of deep breathing and gentle stretches. Slowly, I added positive affirmations, music, and evening walks. These tiny steps restored my spirit, and today I feel more resilient, focused, and vibrant.

1. Navigating Menopause and Other Physical Changes

"Menopause is not an ending. It's a new beginning."

Menopause can feel like a storm—but if navigated mindfully, it leads to a brighter, calmer shore. The hormonal shifts can cause:

✓ Hot flashes and mood swings

✓ Sleep disruptions

✓ Joint pain, fatigue, and memory fog

✓ Weight fluctuations

How to Support Your Body During This Time:

Movement is Medicine: Practice yoga poses like child's pose, cat-cow, or supine twist. Gentle exercises like swimming, walking, or tai chi enhance blood circulation and ease stiffness.

Eat Smart: Include omega-3s (flaxseeds, walnuts), phytoestrogens (soy, sesame), and greens. Avoid too much caffeine or sugar—these worsen symptoms.

Sleep Better: Dim lights before bedtime, sip chamomile tea, or listen to calming audio stories.

Keep Hydrated: Sipping water throughout the day reduces hot flashes and boosts metabolism.

Real-Life Inspiration: Meera, 55, experienced painful joint stiffness during menopause. She was afraid to exercise but began with chair yoga. Over months, with a supportive online yoga coach, she not only regained mobility but also began leading her own community classes from home!

2. Coping with Loneliness, Grief, or Major Life Transitions

"Grief is the price we pay for love."
– Queen Elizabeth II

The transition to an empty nest or losing a loved one can leave a void. Grief may come in waves, but it also opens space to rediscover who you are.

Ways to Heal Emotionally:

Express Yourself: Through journaling, art, poetry, or even voice notes.

Reconnect with Old Passions: Revisit activities that once brought joy—music, crafts, books, prayer, or gardening.

Companionship Matters: Join local senior clubs, spiritual satsangs, or online women's circles.

Seek Support: Therapy or group counseling offers strength through shared experience.

Real Story – Usha's Transformation
Usha, 61, lost her husband unexpectedly. Her world collapsed. But her granddaughter encouraged her to join an online creative writing class. One year later, Usha's short story was published in a regional magazine. "Writing healed me," she says. "It gave me purpose."

3. When to Seek Professional Help (Physical, Mental, and Emotional Well-Being)

"Asking for help doesn't mean you're weak. It means you refuse to give up."

Sometimes we try to "manage" everything. But there's great strength in knowing when to seek professional care.

Watch Out For:

✓ Long-lasting sadness or anger

✓ Isolation or disinterest in daily tasks

✓ Panic attacks or sleepless nights

✓ Loss of appetite or physical aches without cause

Whom to Reach Out To:

- Doctors for physical symptoms, menopause guidance, or chronic fatigue
- Psychologists or counselors for emotional support
- Online apps like InnerHour, Mindhouse, or BetterHelp offer affordable therapy from home

Real Story – Asha's Courage

Asha, 57, began feeling withdrawn and anxious. Her daughter convinced her to speak to a therapist. Over time, Asha found clarity, began volunteering, and now teaches spoken English to underprivileged children—something she had always dreamed of.

4. The Power of Resilience and Adapting to Change

"Resilience is when you face the storm,
not with fear —but with faith."

Life won't always go as planned. But every challenge is an invitation to grow wiser, calmer, and stronger.

Build Resilience By:

- ✓ Gratitude – Write three blessings each morning
- ✓ Learning – Enroll in classes (art, languages, cooking, digital skills)
- ✓ Staying Social – Be part of book clubs, walking groups, or temple gatherings
- ✓ Affirmations – "This too shall pass. I can handle this."

Story: Rekha's Comeback

At 58, Rekha lost her corporate job. Her confidence shattered. But with the support of a friend, she joined a digital marketing course. Today, she works freelance from home and supports her daughter's fashion business. "Setbacks just show you new paths," she says.

Resilience Through Life's Unexpected Challenges

I vividly remember a tough period during my younger daughter's delivery. At the same time, my mother fell seriously ill and was admitted to the ICU in Hyderabad, while my daughter was in Bangalore. Mentally, I was torn. But my mother's strength during that health crisis amazed me. Despite her condition, she radiated calm and hope.

The most inspiring part? She joined me in comforting and energizing my daughter after delivery—her mindset transformed her. From a drained, weak state, she became focused, vibrant, and full of life. Her words of reassurance gave me the courage to manage both sides with grace.

This taught me never to fear situations—face them with a calm mind and open heart. Every challenge carries a solution within it. But in such times, never neglect your health.

Eat nourishing, timely meals. Sleep is essential to feel energetic and balanced. And most importantly, share your emotions. Don't bottle them up. Speak with people who uplift you. Surround yourself with positivity and loving support.

Building Emotional Strength Through Daily Practices

"Every setback we heal from gives us wisdom and glow."

Try These Daily:

- Deep Breathing – The 4-7-8 technique relaxes the nervous system

- Visualization – Close your eyes and picture your vibrant, happiest self
- Morning Affirmations – “I radiate peace. I trust my journey.”
- Nature Therapy – Water your plants, walk barefoot on grass, or feel the morning sun on your face

Inspiring Moment – Sujatha’s Green Oasis

Sujatha, a retired librarian, found joy in terrace gardening. Tending to her tulsi and jasmine plants while humming her favorite bhajans became her healing ritual. “Plants never complain,” she says with a smile. “They just bloom and remind me to do the same.

Cultivating a Sense of Purpose After 50

“You were not born to just do chores —you were born to shine.”

Find Purpose By:

✓ Teaching what you know – cooking, storytelling, singing

✓ Writing your memoir or starting a blog

✓ Volunteering at NGOs or schools

✓ Mentoring young girls or supporting local causes

Example – Shobha’s Zoom Class

Shobha, 62, loved telling stories to her grandchildren. She started a weekly storytelling session over Zoom. Today, children from different cities log in just to hear “Shobha Aunty’s” tales. “It keeps me young and gives the kids a break from screens,” she laughs.

Real-Life Icons Who Inspire

Arunima Sinha – The Unbreakable Spirit

After being thrown from a train and losing her leg, Arunima became the first female amputee to climb Mt. Everest. Her resilience redefined limits and showed the world what true grit looks like.

Sunita Williams – Strength in Orbit

Sunita spent over 286 days in space, navigating intense challenges. Her balance, discipline, and grace under pressure remind us that strength lies in composure and preparation.

Your Resilience Toolkit – Daily Practices to Overcome Setbacks

✓ Gratitude journaling every morning

✓ 10 minutes of joyful movement or yoga

✓ Positive affirmations in the mirror

✓ Nourishing meals at the right time

✓ A heartfelt conversation with a friend

✓ One small act of self-kindness daily

Conclusion: The Comeback Within You

Setbacks are life's way of saying, "Pause. Reflect. Grow." They don't diminish your worth—they reveal your strength.

Whether you're battling joint pain, navigating menopause, grieving a loss, or simply feeling lost—you are not alone. This is your time to rise with grace.

"Every setback is a setup for a greater comeback."

Take a deep breath. Adjust your sails. And remember: the most radiant chapter of your life could begin right now.

■ ■ ■

Chapter 9: Designing Your Fabulous Lifestyle – A Blueprint for Long-Term Success

"Your future is created by what you do today, not tomorrow." – Robert Kiyosaki

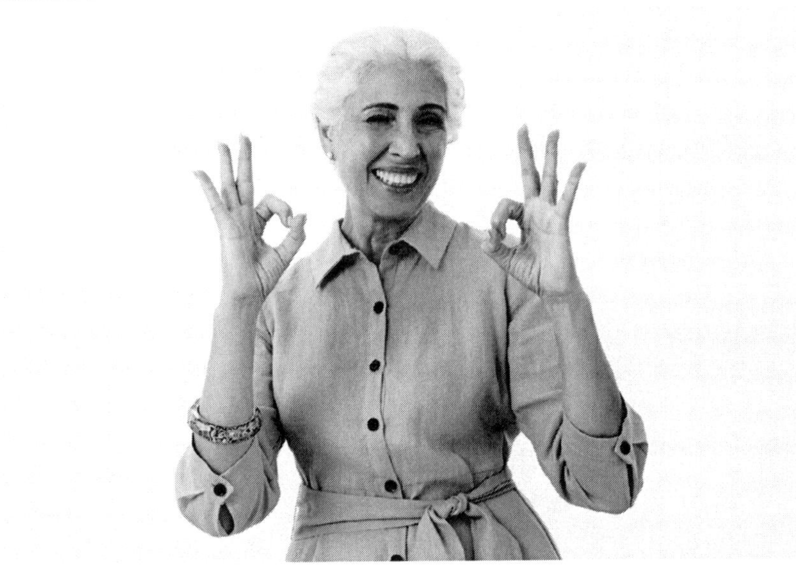

Your Second Act, Your Best Act

Imagine waking up each morning feeling energized, confident, and excited to embrace the day. Picture yourself thriving—not just existing—in this fabulous phase of life. The 50s and beyond are not about slowing down; they're about stepping into a powerful, purposeful version of yourself. This is your time to flourish.

For years, you may have prioritized family, career, and caregiving. Now, it's your turn to prioritize you. The goal of this chapter is to help you create a lifestyle that makes you feel vibrant, fulfilled, and unstoppable—not just for today or tomorrow, but for the years to come.

Let's dive into your personal blueprint for long-term wellness and success: mind, body, and soul.

1. Creating a Sustainable Wellness Plan

"Small habits, when practiced consistently, lead to big transformations."

A sustainable wellness plan is one that fits your lifestyle, aligns with your goals, and feels natural to maintain. It's not about drastic changes—it's about small, meaningful adjustments.

What Should It Include?

✓ **Balanced Nutrition:** Focus on wholesome, seasonal foods. Fresh fruits, vegetables, legumes, nuts, and traditional home-cooked meals can do wonders for energy and digestion.

✓ **Consistent Movement:** Include low-impact activities like yoga, walking, light strength training, and dancing at home.

✓ **Emotional Wellness:** Prioritize self-love, manage stress, and stay socially connected.

✓ **Mental Sharpness:** Keep learning, journaling, and exploring new hobbies.

Example: Rekha's Wellness Shift

Rekha, 55, struggled with energy and motivation. By slowly introducing morning yoga, seasonal fruit bowls, and journaling into her day, she felt a new sense of lightness and control. It wasn't a complete life overhaul—it was a graceful transformation.

Home Exercises You Can Try:

- 10-minute morning stretch
- Wall push-ups
- Seated leg lifts
- Balance practice with a chair
- Gentle evening yoga for relaxation

Nutrition Tip: *Add turmeric, methi, and ginger to your meals for anti-inflammatory benefits. Cook with love, chew slowly, and hydrate generously.*

2. Daily and Weekly Routines to Maintain Vibrancy

"Your habits shape your life more than your decisions."

Routines help bring stability and flow. They create pockets of joy and peace.

Morning Routine

✓ Warm lemon water to detox and energize

✓ 5–10 minutes of prayer or mindfulness

- ✓ Light movement—stretching, yoga, or a walk
- ✓ A protein-rich breakfast like dal chilla or ragi porridge
- ✓ Positive affirmations like: "I radiate energy and joy."

Evening Routine

- ✓ Unwind with herbal tea or golden milk
- ✓ Disconnect from screens by 8:00 PM
- ✓ Light reading, music, or breathing exercises
- ✓ Gratitude journaling: 3 wins from the day

Real-Life Example: Radha's Daily Glow

Radha, 52, shifted from chaotic mornings to structured days with gentle habits. Within weeks, her sleep improved, mood lifted, and her skin glowed.

3. Setting Goals and Celebrating Progress

"A goal without a plan is just a wish."
– Antoine de Saint-Exupéry

Why Set Goals After 50? Because goals give you direction, purpose, and a reason to stay inspired.

Use the SMART Formula:

- ✓ Specific: Write down exactly what you want to do.
- ✓ Measurable: Track your progress weekly.
- ✓ Achievable: Start small to build confidence.
- ✓ Relevant: Choose what aligns with your life.

✓ Time-bound: Set realistic deadlines.

Suman's 60-Day Challenge

Suman, 54, set a goal to walk 5,000 steps daily and meditate for 5 minutes. She tracked it using a journal. After 60 days, she lost 4 kgs, felt calmer, and started inspiring other women in her community.

Celebrate Small Wins:

✓ Pamper yourself with a spa at home

✓ Share your achievement in your friend circle

✓ Light a diya to celebrate progress

4. Living with Purpose and Excitement for the Future

"The meaning of life is to give life meaning."

Purpose fuels energy. When we do what we love, age disappears.

Finding Purpose After 50

✓ What brings you joy? Dancing, writing, singing, gardening?

✓ How can you give back? Mentor younger women, teach skills online

✓ What dream did you put on hold? Now is the time to reignite it.

Real-Life Achievers Who Started Late

Arunima Sinha – After losing her leg in a train accident, she became the first female amputee to climb Mount Everest. Her courage is a reminder that limitations are only in the mind.

Harbhajan Kaur – At 90, she started selling home-made sweets. Her daughter supported her, and soon she became a household name in Chandigarh.

Neelam Saxena Chandra – A poet and railway officer, she started publishing books in her 50s and now inspires women writers across India.

5. Nourishment for Body and Mind – At Home Nutrition & Mental Care

Nutrition Habits That Energize:

✓ Seasonal fruits like guava, papaya, and berries

✓ Ragi, bajra, and whole grains for strength

✓ Green leafy vegetables thrice a week

✓ Herbal teas—tulsi, chamomile, ginger

✓ Healthy snacks—roasted chana, nuts, yogurt with flaxseeds

Mind Nourishment Practices:

✓ Journaling: Write thoughts, dreams, and wins

✓ Affirmations: Repeat phrases like "I am enough," "I am strong"

✓ Visualization: Close your eyes and imagine your best self

✓ Reading motivational literature

✓ Light crossword puzzles, Sudoku, and memory games

6. Social Wellness – Building and Nurturing Your Tribe

"Surround yourself with those who lift you higher."

Stay Connected:

✓ Join WhatsApp learning groups

✓ Create weekly Zoom catch-ups with cousins or friends

✓ Volunteer at local NGOs or online storytelling clubs

✓ Form a hobby group in your apartment complex

Real-Life Example:

Shobha, 62, created a "Golden Circle" group where women gather weekly to learn something new. From digital skills to healthy recipes, they grow together.

Your Fabulous Lifestyle Blueprint – Action Plan

✓ Design a joyful morning and evening routine

✓ Set one 30-day SMART goal

✓ Try a new healthy recipe each week

✓ Join a community or group that excites you

✓ Move your body daily (even 10 minutes)

✓ Practice journaling or mindfulness daily

✓ Celebrate your wins and reflect regularly

✓ Practice 3 deep breaths every time you feel overwhelmed

Conclusion: Your Best Life Begins Now

Designing your fabulous lifestyle is not a luxury—it's your right. You have walked through decades of love, work, joy, and challenges. Now, you walk into a future filled with purpose, strength, and elegance.

This chapter—and this book—isn't the end of your story. It's the start of your most radiant one.

"The best time to plant a tree was 20 years ago.
The second-best time is now."

Start today. Create habits that nurture you. Seek joy in the ordinary. Build rituals that celebrate your worth. Because the most fabulous woman you'll ever become—is already within you.

Shine on.

■ ■ ■

Chapter 10: Your Best Years Are Now – A Powerful Conclusion to Your Fabulous Journey

"Do not go where the path may lead, go instead where there is no path and leave a trail."
– Ralph Waldo Emerson

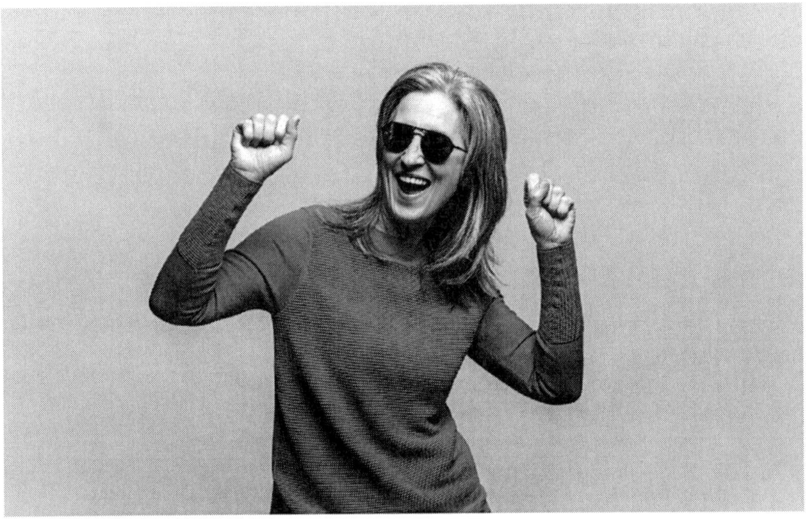

1. Reflecting on Your Journey

A Celebration of the Journey

You've made it. You've read through the nine empowering chapters of this book, and hopefully, you've begun to rediscover the incredible woman you are—vibrant, wise, strong, and full of untapped potential. The journey we've taken together was never just about fitness or food or routines. It was about you—your dreams, your growth, and your spirit.

Now, in this final chapter, we bring it all together into a vision for your most radiant, resilient, and joyful life ahead.

Rewind, Reflect, Reignite

Let's briefly revisit what we've discovered in the previous chapters, each offering you a gift:

Chapter 1 reminded you that 50 is not a finish line but a new, exciting starting point. Through mindset shifts and self-belief, you learned to embrace joy and growth.

Chapter 2 made you move—not just physically, but emotionally. You saw how simple movement can reignite energy, relieve pain, and restore vitality.

Chapter 3 brought you back to the power of nourishment, not just to fill your stomach, but to fuel your body and mind for long-lasting energy and youthfulness.

Chapter 4 taught you to recognize and release stress, making room for peace through practices like mindfulness, self-care, and joyful routines.

Chapter 5 helped you reclaim beauty on your own terms—through confidence, elegance, and embracing your unique style and natural glow.

Chapter 6 showed how staying mentally sharp is not only possible but invigorating—learning new skills, exploring passions, and keeping curiosity alive.

Chapter 7 emphasized connection—how circles of support, online communities, and friendship keep your spirit uplifted and your life meaningful.

Chapter 8 gave you the courage to rise from setbacks—through stories of resilience, healing, and the power of hope.

Chapter 9 gave you the blueprint to build a fabulous lifestyle—sustainable, joyful, and rooted in purpose and excitement for the future.

2. A Call to Action: Keep Moving, Keep Glowing, Keep Thriving

---

Designing Your "New Normal"

You are not here just to survive the years ahead—you are here to design them with intention, color, and power.

1. Live with Energy – Physical Wellness at Home

Daily Practices:

✓ Stretch every morning to wake your body.

✓ Walk for 20 minutes—even in your home corridor or on your terrace.

✓ Practice simple chair yoga or dance while listening to your favorite music.

✓ Try resistance band workouts to build strength safely.

✓ Hydrate—start your day with warm water and lemon, and sip water throughout the day.

Real-Life Inspiration: Pushpa, 62, a homemaker from Bengaluru, reversed her pre-diabetic condition by walking 30 minutes every morning, switching to millet-based meals, and practicing yoga at home using YouTube videos. Today, she radiates energy and mentors other women in her neighborhood.

2. Fuel Your Body – Simple Nutrition That Heals

Smart Tips:

✓ Start your day with protein—eggs, sprouts, or moong dal cheela.

✓ Add leafy greens, seeds (flax, chia), and seasonal fruits to your meals.

✓ Limit refined sugar—use jaggery, dates, or fruits instead.

✓ Have dinner early and light for better sleep and digestion.

✓ Sip turmeric milk, herbal teas (tulsi, chamomile) in the evening.

Recipe to Try: Ragi Porridge with Almond Milk and Banana – full of calcium and iron, this is a brain and bone booster.

3. Build Resilience – Emotional Wellness & Mindset

Empowering Practices:

✓ Affirmations: "I am strong. I am enough. I am becoming the best version of myself."

✓ Journal your thoughts—release emotional clutter, reflect and heal.

✓ Mindfulness walks—observe your surroundings with all your senses.

✓ Celebrate small wins—applaud yourself for taking action.

Real-Life Story: Urmila, 57, lost her spouse unexpectedly. Through journaling, volunteering at a children's library, and attending spiritual satsangs, she found healing and a new sense of meaning.

4. Ignite Your Mind – Cognitive & Creative Strength

Try These:

- ✓ Learn something new—languages, music, painting, or digital tools.
- ✓ Read motivational books—"The Power of Now," "Atomic Habits," "Big Magic."
- ✓ Join a book club or online learning circle.
- ✓ Practice memory games, puzzles, and impromptu speech challenges.

Inspiring Woman: Lakshmi, 65, began learning piano at home and now performs devotional music in small gatherings, proving passion never retires.

5. Connect Deeply – Social & Spiritual Bonding

Ways to Stay Connected:

- ✓ Call one friend daily—just to chat and laugh.
- ✓ Celebrate festivals with family, cook together, share stories.
- ✓ Join WhatsApp or Zoom groups for hobbies or wellness.
- ✓ Volunteer—even small acts of kindness fuel the soul.
- ✓ Practice gratitude prayer or chant for 5 minutes each morning.

6. Leave a Legacy – Live with Purpose

- ✓ Mentor younger women—share your life lessons.
- ✓ Start a home business or blog—your passion may inspire many.
- ✓ Write your story—leave behind your journey for future generations.

Example: Raji, 59, started recording voice messages of her life lessons for her grandkids. Her children turned them into a podcast that now inspires women around the world.

Action Plan: Your Fabulous Future Starts Today

Let's make it tangible. Tick these off over the next 30 days:

- ✓ Wake up with gratitude
- ✓ Move for at least 15 minutes
- ✓ Eat one colorful, home-cooked meal
- ✓ Call or message a friend
- ✓ Do one joyful activity (music, painting, dancing)
- ✓ Learn or read something new
- ✓ Affirm yourself aloud
- ✓ Smile at your reflection
- ✓ Sleep for 7–8 hours
- ✓ Plan tomorrow with ex

3. Final Words of Encouragement

"It is never too late to be what you might have been."
– George Eliot

Dear Fabulous Woman,

You have loved, lost, created, sacrificed, and dreamed. You have shown strength in silence, courage in chaos, and grace in growth.

Now it's your time—to shine, to soar, to sparkle.

Don't wait for the perfect time. Don't shrink because of fear or age. Dance, laugh, fall in love with life again. Let your 50s and beyond be a masterpiece—not of perfection, but of passion.

Your best years are not ahead. They are now—waiting for you to live them fully.

Stay strong. Stay radiant. Stay fabulous.

■ ■ ■